Women Over 40's Bodybuilding Diet:

A Complete Guide to Reaching Your Fitness Objectives, Discover the Techniques for Gaining Strength, Losing Fat, and Defying your Exercises

Susan M. Burnnet

All rights reserved. No part of this publication may be reproduced, distributed, or transmitted in any form or by any means, including photocopying, recording, or other electronic or mechanical methods, without the prior written permission of the publisher, except in the case of brief quotations embodied in critical reviews and certain other noncommercial uses permitted by copyright law.

Copyright © (Susan M. Burnnet), (2023).

Table of Content

Chapter One

The Fundamentals of Bodybuilding for Female above 40 years

The ultimate in bodybuilding competition attire, if you decide to partake in the sport, is undoubtedly the most dazzling bikini you have ever laid eyes on. However, being a female bodybuilder has a lot less glamorous side as well: food planning and dieting, tracking macros, getting up early to work out, spending hours in the weight room, and scraping off calluses on your hands.

Lifting weights has many health advantages, but bodybuilding "does not come without its fair share of sacrifice, if this is your passion, it's worth every second. "You must use your mental toughness and willpower to achieve the empowering gains in bodybuilding, which will benefit all aspects of your life.

How Does Bodybuilding Work?

In actuality, bodybuilding in sport comes with a very strict way of living that includes exact eating and exercise regimens to build, tone, and grow the body muscles (also known as hypertrophy training).

While some individuals bodybuild for the sake of feeling and looking strong, for many, the end goal of their training and dieting is to compete in a bodybuilding competition where their muscular growth and appearance is evaluated in one of the following categories: fitness, bodybuilding, figure, bikini, or women's physique.

Before you continue, be aware that playing a sport where your physical appearance is your primary source of evaluation might have a negative psychological impact. Together with your physical health, it is important to take care of your soul and mind. As one expert put it, "If you already struggle with body image issues, attaining what the outside world (or judges) views as the perfect aesthetic does not guarantee that you will see a different person in the mirror."

A physique competition may be a terrific method to focus your strength training goals, but remember that the improvements you're making in terms of your health and performance are more significant than the judges' assessment of your abs.

That being said, even if your goal is just to gain strength and you have no desire to compete, you may still benefit from bodybuilding routines and the training approach.

Plans for Female Bodybuilding Exercises

How can one develop amazing muscular mass with regular strength training?

Regular bodybuilding exercise is difficult, it usually involves training twice a day — approximately one hour of lifting and anywhere from 30 minutes to two hours of cardio per day.

A normal 5-day split would be like this: The majority of female bodybuilders plan their workouts by allocating their strength training days according to certain body parts, a practice known as a "split."

Day 1: torso

Day 2: Returning

Day 3: Arms

Day 4: Lower Body

Day 5: Weapons

Days 6 and 7: Leisure time

That being said, each person's exercise regimen will vary somewhat based on their objectives and body type. "Most lifters schedule their work so that they concentrate on one body area each day, but you may alternate between legs and upper body exercises every three days.

A common preference among athletes is to work out each muscle group twice a week. To do this, you may plan your training such that you alternate between a leg exercise day, a "pull" day, and a "push" day.

Day 1: Push your triceps, shoulders, and chest.

Day 2: Biceps and back pulls

Day 3: Lower Body

Day 4: Push your triceps, shoulders, and chest.

Day 5: Biceps and back pulls

Day 6: Lower Body

Day 7: Unwind

After warming up, you should usually execute three to five exercises for the targeted body area, completing three to four sets of eight to twelve repetitions for each.

It is a good idea to begin with complex exercises (i.e., exercises that utilise many joints, like squats, bench presses, deadlifts, etc.) and progress to isolation exercises (i.e., exercises that use a single joint, like leg extensions and bicep curls).

Isolation exercises are important for bodybuilding workouts because they focus on one muscle at a time and are effective in increasing the size of muscle fibres, which is a major goal of all bodybuilders.

Additionally, if you're new to strength training, these simpler exercises will help keep you moving safely and injury-free. Compound exercises usually get all the glory because they allow you to hoist bigger weights and count as functional training.

You should only be operating at 60–70% of your one repetition maximum (ORM) while doing 8–12 repetitions of each exercise.

"Building strength and power is best achieved by lifting closer to 100% of your 1RM, but bodybuilders are more concerned with muscle size," "It is preferable to lift for longer durations in order to cause hypertrophy, or an increase in muscle size." Bodybuilders often use less weight for more repetitions because of this."

Supersets, which are essentially two exercises that target the same muscle group back-to-back, frequently with little to no rest in between, are another useful training technique. Tempo is also important, as you want to lift very slowly and controlled throughout the entire range of motion. All of these techniques are effective in producing muscle fatigue and microtears in the muscle fibres, which the body repairs during rest, causing the muscle fibres to grow back thicker, leading to hypertrophy, or an increase in muscle size."

Indeed, aerobic exercise is necessary. "Cardio is crazy important!". Aim for 20 minutes of cardio three times a week. "This will help uncover the beautiful muscular shape you're creating."

How Women Can Begin Bodybuilding

Employ a coach: Hiring a coach is something you should do without a doubt. However, don't settle for someone who seems nice on **Instagram**: "You're putting them in charge of your health, so it's important to do a lot of research so that you find a coach who can guide you with a good training and nutrition plan."

Log everything: "Make sure you log your training so you can strategically increase your weights over time." (Some of these food tracking apps can help you monitor all that in one place on your quest to become a female bodybuilder.) It's also very helpful to log your food so you can keep track of your macros and calories.

Remember to use machines: "If you're new to bodybuilding but have a good strength base, go ahead and play with the free weights. These typically engage more muscles that help stabilise the body throughout an exercises range of motion." "For beginner weightlifters, using machines can be beneficial as these keep the body in the proper place throughout the exercise."

Give yourself lots of time: If you want to compete, provide enough time to prepare and gain muscle. You won't need to take long to prepare if you're more consistent with your nutrition and training, especially during your off-season. "Everyone is different, but new competitors are typically ready to compete after a 12-week intensive period."

There is a method to bodybuilding, "it is progressive in nature and requires a customised plan," but be patient. It will keep you safe and be effective and efficient when executed correctly. However, building bigger and stronger muscles requires persistence, patience, and work. Biceps and glutes don't develop overnight.

Continue to raise the bar: "As with any other training programme, your body will adapt, so it's crucial to test yourself regularly to make sure that you are adjusting the weights, reps, and/or the amount of rest in between sets properly as you get stronger to maintain or even increase the intensity of the workouts"

Advantages of bodybuilding for women who are over 40

Although there isn't always equal representation or opportunity for men and women in the bodybuilding field, it's important to include extreme weight lifting into your lifestyle since it may have major health advantages for women.

Although bodybuilding requires a significant commitment, it's a worthwhile endeavour. Fortunately, women bodybuilding has been extensively studied by others, and many beginner bodybuilding principles have been put to the test and shown to be applicable to both genders.

We would guide you through the fitness advantages of bodybuilding for women in this book, explaining specific exercise regimens, suggested diets, and much more.

Advantages of female bodybuilding for fitness. (Women Bodybuilding Exercise Benefits)

Developed and Enhanced Bone Density

Regular resistance exercise or weight training promotes bone development and raises total bone mineral density; medical research clearly shows that postmenopausal women face a decrease of bone density.

Enhanced Metabolism

Increased muscle mass helps your body burn more calories even when it is at rest. The more muscle mass you have, the more calories your body will burn, the more calories you burn, the thinner you will become. Moreover, increased muscle mass will give your body more definition and reduce the amount of fat that has accumulated in certain areas of your body.

More Robust Joints

Ligament injuries are more common in women than in men. Exercises used in bodybuilding, such as lunges and squats, strengthen the muscles that support the hips and other joints.

Better Posture, Mobility, and Balance

These advantages come from a combination of stronger hips and legs, more developed bone density, and increased upper-body strength. They may also help prevent shoulder and back injuries, which would improve posture and balance.

Improved Mood

Bodybuilding workouts help with better sleep, increased energy levels, and a sense of accomplishment. Since women are twice as likely as men to develop clinical depression, working out helps combat mood swings due to the release of naturally occurring mood-enhancing chemicals like dopamine, serotonin, and norepinephrine.

Modification of Macronutrients

A diet that contains 80% of calories from carbohydrates, 10% from protein, and 10% from fat will produce different results than a diet that contain 40% of calories from carbohydrates, 40% from protein, and 20% from fat. Therefore, maintaining a personalised balanced diet as per your individual health and fitness goal is very essential for fitness in women bodybuilding. The ratio of protein to carbs to fat can determine whether the weight you gain or lose is actually muscle or fat.

Maintain Hydration

We all know that drinking lots of water is good for us in general and for our daily lives. Aim for eight glasses (64 oz.) or more per day, as this will provide you optimal hydration and a feeling of fullness without adding calories. Since people sometimes confuse thirst for hunger, drinking water can also help you avoid overeating.

Adequate Protein

In order to gain lean muscle mass, you need to eat enough protein to sustain the development of new muscles. You may not be used to eating the number of proteins prescribed by dietitians in the beginning, once you get used to the diet and workout, you will enjoy how full and satisfied you will feel with a balanced diet and regular workout routine.

Essential Fats Essential fatty acids are vital to the proper functioning of your body; a certain amount of fat content is needed by the body and is definitely a part of a healthy diet. Many essential fatty acids help support the fat-burning process and maintaining a lean body. Make sure to follow your nutritionist/dietitians for good fat intake.

Choosing the correct form of exercise

As you get older, you can't just Blaze, Cyclone or Whirlwind. Like you used to in your 20's and 30's without risk of injury or exhaustion. As you age, your body responds differently to exercise depending on factors like diet, lifestyle, hormone balance, genetics, mobility and general health.

In your 40's and beyond, it's not a matter of simply 'eat less, exercise more'! This approach may be counter productive since it might stress your body out instead of feeding it.

Exercise is crucial for hormones and overall health as it improves stress levels, sleep quality, mood, brain health and insulin function. And if you go beyond 40, it is the ideal moment to pursue a more balanced and potentially a more sustainable approach to exercise.

Workout for Women over 40

These are my top ideas for women over 40 to consider putting in your routine. You don't have to do them all, there are many other things you could love more (like jogging, skiing, dancing or whatever you're into). It's just to start you thinking of what your body needs.

1. Resistance & Weights

this one is placed first for a reason — strength training is one of the finest shields against the affects of ageing! Which is why I'm now taking this one seriously on a personal level.

Not only can exercise help counteract the muscular mass we lose as we grow older, boosting the metabolism and lowering fat deposits, but it may also enhance mental health and mood, and lessen the danger of accidents.

Strength training also increases bone density, hence minimising your chance of osteoporosis, a major worry for many of us as we approach towards our menopausal years.

Strength training may be included into your programme in a variety of ways, such as utilising a park bench as a tri-cep dip stop or keeping some weights or resistance bands in your workout gear at home. It's the holy grail of fitness for women over 40, and I want you to benefit from it as much as possible.

Enhance your resistance and weight training regimen by enrolling in a body pump or kettlebell class and gradually increasing the weights.

2. Make NEAT function for you.

This isn't exactly an exercise kind, but it's a very important kind of movement. Sitting is a big health concern these days, but there are some simple changes we can make to our daily routine to lessen its negative effects on our health and hormones. We can do this by increasing our NEAT (Non Exercise

Activity Thermogenesis) activity by doing small but daily acts of supercharge.

Invest in a standing desk, balancing ball, or both in place of a chair. This is a top NEAT suggestion since it may significantly minimise your amount of time spent static sitting and increase your NEAT potential.

3. Walk and Talk

Did you know that therapists are now consulting in the closest park instead of the consultation room? This is because, as nature surrounds us, we tend to have the finest discussions. I know that when I'm walking, I always come up with my best ideas.

Give yourself permission to take frequent breaks; you'll be less stressed and more productive in the long term. Just consider how much 5–10 minutes of exercise per hour adds up— it's like squeezing in an additional hour of exercise every day without even realising it!

Boost your resistance training: dumbbells next to the kettle so you can get in a little power workout while it's heating up.

4. Strolling

There aren't many things that can revitalise you like going for a vigorous walk and taking a deep breath of fresh air. Walking has several health advantages, ranging from reducing your risk of chronic illness to elevating your mood.

Therefore, if none of the other suggestions appeal to you, try "just walking", adding a few walks to your weekly routine could be exactly what the doctor ordered. Additionally, as long as you don't have an injury, there are essentially no barriers to entry because it's simple, affordable, and convenient.

Incorporate resistance training by using weighted jackets or wrist and ankle weights, and increase the number of walks you do on steep terrain.

5. HIIT

Try HIIT, or "High Intensity Interval Training," if your joints are in good condition, your stress level is manageable, and you're in good health. Studies have shown that HIIT burns fat more efficiently than aerobic exercise.

In terms of the body ability to acquire strength, HIIT exercises have not only been shown to do so faster than more conventional resistance training, but in some instances, they have also been shown to increase strength gains above traditional resistance training.

There are no longer excuses for not having time to workout since it is made to be very time-efficient. So why wait?

6. **Supercharge with resistance:**

No need! Three times a week, 15 minutes is all that's needed to get going.

7. **Diving**

For women over forty, swimming is an excellent kind of non-weight bearing cardiovascular exercise that works the whole body. It is essentially helpful for those of us who still want to feel good about our bodies but are experiencing joint difficulties as we age. Good news for our hormones as well a 2016 research with 62 untrained perimenopausal women revealed that swimming three times a week increased insulin sensitivity and glycemic management.

If you want to undertake high-intensity interval training (HIIT) but are hesitant because you fear your joints will not handle it, consider trying low-volume, high-intensity intermittent swimming instead of swimming at a low intensity for an hour. You may also benefit from cold exposure, which is known to be very beneficial to health, by going for a wild swim in the outdoors.

8. Boost your workout with resistance

If you're stuck in the pool, try arm or leg floats, paddles, tethers, or, if you're feeling really daring, a bouy!

9. Pilates & Yoga

The finest forms of exercise for women over 40 are yoga and pilates, which provide several advantages including improved flexibility, strength, posture, less stress, and improved mood.

Finding the time to sit in a quiet room and think about nothing for ten minutes can feel indulgent, even boring for many. However, yoga and pilates give you that time to be present; focusing on the pose and your breathing. A calming tonic for our stressful daily lives. Being mindful is such a buzz word and to some it may feel totally unattainable.

There are lots of options available, so try out a couple and play about until you discover one you really like.

10. **Supercharge with resistance**

A decent yoga session will be plenty. If you want to take a Pilates Reformer class, these are wonderful for really targeting certain muscle regions.

11. **Core and Pelvic Floor Strength**

It is not acceptable to ignore your pelvic floor and core, particularly if you have children, so be sure to include this into your regimen.

When it comes to protecting the pelvic floor and preventing any "oops" moments that may occur when you cough or sneeze, Kegel exercises are the best.

Kegels are great because, once you get the hang of them, you can do them whenever you have a few seconds to spare, including while waiting for a bus, standing in queue at a photocopier or riding in an elevator.

12. One word of warning though

Take the time to get the fundamentals right and get advice from a pelvic floor specialist or physiotherapist if you are concerned. Up to one-third of women do the exercises improperly because of bad posture or inappropriate breathing, which merely adds to the stress.

Within six weeks of mastering the method, set aside a few minutes many times a day, and you should see a change.

To develop and identify your pelvic floor muscles, use Kegel balls for specific workout. This will help you supercharge with resistance.

Myths Concerning Female Bodybuilding

The most pervasive fallacy about women's bodybuilding and/or fitness is that they must spend hours doing cardio exercises to retain their "feminine" shape since doing too much weight training would make them seem strong and masculine.

That being said, women's testosterone levels are a fraction of men's, so weight training will not make women look more masculine. As a woman who follows weight training for fitness, such an outcome is highly unlikely. The truth is that women lack the hormonal support that men have to gain muscle mass.

As much as everyone would want to be able to eat everything they want, we all should know that it doesn't work that way! Another frequent fallacy that people like to think, particularly women, is that you can eat whatever you want provided you're exercising to burn it away.

You just need to use restraint; if you overindulge in dessert, forget about it and move on. You don't need to punish yourself by doing extra cardio to burn those calories, as it won't work and will only create an unhealthy relationship with food and exercise. Exercise does burn calories, but not nearly enough to make up for bingeing on whatever strikes your fancy.

Chapter Two

Diet for Bodybuilding

It's been said that because of better healthier behaviours, 40 is the new 30. However, when they approach their 40s, women (like men) still battle with weight and other health issues.

At this age, your body's requirements for nutrition (food and water) and metabolism (the rate at which food is turned into energy) vary. Your rate of metabolism decreases. Women begin to lose almost half a pound of muscle a year after turning forty. That increases the difficulty of reducing weight. Women go through many changes, some of which are brought on by low hormone levels, low levels of exercise, and illnesses.

Way to achieve more healthy diet

As you get closer to forty years old, diet becomes increasingly more crucial. Women need nutritious grains for carbs, healthy oils for fats, fish, meat, beans, and nuts for protein, as well as vitamins, minerals, and water. various meals have been associated with the prevention of various diseases, including high blood pressure, diabetes, heart disease, osteoporosis, and certain types of cancer. To increase the availability of healthy food, the American Academy of Family Physicians advocates the creation of supply chains for healthy foods in supplementary nutrition programmes.

Nourishment

By the time you become forty, if you haven't started taking your nutrition seriously, now is the moment. Select both starchy and non-starchy veggies, as well as dark green, red, and orange beans and peas.

Consume a range of fruits

Make grains a part of your diet every day. You should eat whole grains for half of your diet. Opt for low-fat or fat-free dairy products. Milk, yogurt, cheese, and fortified soy products fall within this category. Consume protein with every meal. Lean meat (chicken), fish, eggs, beans and peas, nuts, seeds, and soy products are good sources of protein. Make use of healthful oils like olive oil.

Furthermorwoman need to eat:

-   Less than 10% of your daily calories which come from processed meals and sweets that have added sugar.

-   Less than 10% of daily calories come which from high-fat dairy and red meat.

-   Not more than 2,300 mg of salt per day

-   Limiting alcohol consumption to one drink each day

-   Calcium, potassium, dietary fibre, vitamin A, and vitamin

The value of a balanced diet

A well-balanced diet doesn't have to be difficult. You will be well on your way to a healthier life if you heed the advice of experts and eat a balanced diet. Making appropriate dietary adjustments to help control your weight, avoid illness, and improve your overall well-being is something you should do at any time of the day. Here are some benefits of a balanced diet for your well-being.

A Balanced Diet:
What Is It?

A balanced diet consists of a range of foods from various food groups, namely: fruits and vegetables; dairy products (low-fat milk, cheese, yoghurt); meat, fish, eggs, beans, and soy; carbs (starchy foods like rice, pasta, potatoes, and bread, preferably wholegrain or wholewheat varieties); and a small number of healthy fats (like the unsaturated fat from olive oil). Steer clear of sugary beverages and meals, as well as processed meats, chips, pies, and pastries that have additional saturated fat. To stay hydrated and support improved bodily functions, drink plenty of water.

What Advantages Does a Balanced Diet Offer?

Stops infections and illnesses

Your immune system is strengthened when you consume the whole spectrum of vitamins, minerals, and other nutrients. A nutritious diet may even help ward against illnesses like cancer, heart disease, diabetes, and stroke.

Assists you in managing your weight Eating a balanced diet helps you regulate your weight and maintain it over time. Most individuals wish to gain or lose weight at some point. A balanced diet is the only way to maintain long-term, healthful weight control—weight reduction diets are not sustainable.

Enhances mental well-being It is important to take care of yourself by eating healthily while you work towards excellent mental health. Getting the correct balance of nutrients may help reduce the symptoms of anxiety and sadness.

Good for growth

A well-balanced diet is essential for kids and teenagers. To ensure that cells are formed and maintained and that the body develops at the proper rate, the body must get the proper nutrients while it expands.

Improved hair and skin

A well-balanced diet enhances your appearance as well. Eating a balanced diet helps you appear younger by promoting good skin and hair.

TIMING OF NUTRIENTS FOR RECOVERY

Making sure your pre-exercise meal(s) sufficiently fuels your activity and optimizing your macronutrients, as previously discussed, to maintain glycogen storage and protein balance, are important aspects of timing your nutrition for recovery.

Although the post-exercise "optimal window" is a topic of controversy, it is believed that optimising adaptations and recovery and minimising adrenal stress and catabolism may be achieved by replenishing glycogen and consuming protein shortly after exercise or an event.

SUMMARY FOR RECOVERY

Only until the foundation (energy, macros, micros, hydration, and timing) is addressed can supplements aid in enhancing healing. Supplements may be divided into groups according to how they aid in bone, tendon, and muscle healing as well as how they promote inflammation rather than inhibit it.

inflammatory response

Inflammatory Response

- **Bromelain**: Usually 500 mg three times a day, away from food
- **Curcumin**: 500 mg three times a day (look for a piperidine-containing product)

Fish oil: 2000 mg three times a day

Repairing Muscle

Sufficient protein (refer to the protein section)

Beta-hydroxy-beta-methyl butyrate (HMB): 3 grams per day

- 4000 mg/day of fish oil
- Creatine Monohydrate: split dosages of 5000 mg/day for five days, then 3000 mg/day
- Polyphenols: Incorporate a range of vibrant fruits, vegetables, herbs, and spices into your diet to get these micronutrients from plant-based foods. Studies have shown that tart

cherry juice may help with pain and muscle regeneration.

Tendon Restoration:

• Gelatin or collagen: 10g daily

• Whey Protein: 20–40 g daily, of which 3-5 g are leucine.

• Nitrates: Found in foods like chard and beets, they promote circulation

• Citrulline malate: 6,000–8,000 mg/day: promotes blood flow

Bone Mending:

Sufficient Protein and Carbohydrate Intake

- Calcium: Consume 1200 mg of calcium, mostly from food.

- Vitamin D: Based on blood testing, 40–60 ng/mL are ideal values.

- Smoothie for recuperation; about two servings

- One cup of water

- One cup of spinach or greens
- One peeled beetroot
- ½ cup organic frozen berries
- One banana
- Half an avocado
- Tsp raw cacao
- 30 grames of whey protein
- 2 tablespoons ground flaxseed

Mix things and savor!

Muscular Mass

If you want to gain strength and increase your muscular mass, consider the following:

Sufficient protein intake is necessary for the ideal diet for growing muscle. Aim for 1.7 to 1.8 grams of protein per kilogramme of bodyweight per day for women who strength train.3 A 140-pound woman (63.6 kg) would have roughly 115 grams of protein daily. More precisely, this protein has to come from meals high in complete protein, such as those derived from dairy and meat from animals, or complete vegetarian sources, such as hemp or peas. Because only necessary amino acids, which are plentiful in complete protein, drive muscle protein synthesis and prevent breakdown, complete protein sources are crucial.

The only way to gain muscle is via intense strength training. Muscle protein synthesis is stimulated during the post-exercise phase, but this is not enough to counteract the accompanying muscle loss. This is where eating a healthy diet is important. Strength exercise helps repair and create muscle protein, which leads to muscular hypertrophy (muscle development). It works in concert with an ideal calorie and protein diet.

Since the focus of this book is on nutritional considerations for muscle hypertrophy, I will not go into great detail about resistance training here. Instead, I will emphasize the significance of dietary protein, the effects of getting enough calories and carbs, and the benefits of taking creatine supplements as these are important factors that support muscle growth.

What Amount of Protein Is Needed?

The optimal amount of protein required for the production of muscle protein has been studied. Historically, males have been the subjects of the bulk of these studies. Men may require more protein than women because, according to scant research on the subject, men oxidize (burn) more amino acids during exercise and at rest.5 Since reliable data on women's protein needs is scarce, you are free to either strictly adhere to these recommendations or make adjustments in light of your own experiences.

Regarding total protein intake, the recommendation of 1.7 to 1.8 grams per kilogramme of body weight per day seems to apply fairly accurately to women.[3,4] Some people believe that consuming even more protein is even more beneficial, but studies have shown that the maximum amount of protein that can be used to build muscle is 2.0 grams per kilogramme per day.[7] The advantages of consuming more protein in the diet go beyond muscle hypertrophy.

Since protein burns more calories during a meal than fats or carbs, it may aid in increasing caloric expenditure. When total calorie intake is not excessive, protein is less likely to be stored as body fat than fats or carbs and is more satiating, which helps manage desire. While protein may be utilised as fuel in cases when fats and carbs are not well tolerated, it is not as effective as protein as an energy source for working out muscles. Since protein converts to glucose more slowly than carbs, it may help avoid blood sugar spikes and falls.

Recommended macronutrient ratio

Your body needs macronutrients—carbohydrates, lipids, and proteins—in huge quantities. According to a study, eating habits may have a greater impact on weight reduction than dietary intake of carbohydrates, fats, and proteins.

Macronutrient counting has been a recent fad in weight reduction. These are the nutrients—carbs, lipids, and proteins—that your body needs in substantial quantities for proper growth and development. Conversely, micronutrients—such as vitamins and minerals—are those that your body only needs in trace quantities. While calculating calories and macronutrients are similar, macronutrient counting takes into account the source of calories.

This book discusses why diet quality is important and what macronutrient ratio is ideal for weight reduction.

For fat loss, calorie intake is more important than the ratio of macronutrients. Throughout 600 overweight participants were randomized to a low-fat or low-carb diet throughout a year-long trial.

The low-fat diet group consumed 20 grams of fat per day and the low-carb group received 20 grams of carbohydrates per day throughout the first two months of the trial.
Following two months, participants in both groups started reintroducing either fats or carbohydrates into their diets until they

achieved the lowest quantity they thought they could sustain.

Both groups cut their daily caloric intake by an average of 500–600 calories, although neither group was required to eat a certain amount of calories.

The low-carb group dropped 13.2 pounds (6 kg) after the research, whereas the low-fat diet group lost 11.7 pounds (5.3 kg)—a difference of just 1.5 pounds (0.7 kg) over a year.

Over two years, all diets were similarly effective in inducing identical levels of weight reduction, regardless of the macronutrient ratio. These and other findings suggest that any diet with fewer calories may, over time, result in comparable levels of weight reduction.

Note: A calorie is a unit of measurement for the energy content of a certain meal or drink. One food calorie, whether it comes from fats, proteins, or carbohydrates, has around 4.2 joules of energy in it.

It follows that all calories are equal under this definition. This presumption, however, ignores the complexity of human physiology.
Your metabolic rate, hormonal reaction, and level of hunger or fullness may all be influenced by food and its macronutrient makeup of it

Therefore, even if 100 calories from broccoli and 100 calories from doughnuts provide the same amount of energy, they have quite distinct effects on your body and dietary choices.
Seven grams of fibre and almost 100 calories may be found in three cups (270 grams) of raw broccoli. On the other hand, two doughnut holes have little more than 100 calories, mostly from processed carbohydrates and fats.

Imagine now if you could have four cups of broccoli at once. Its high fibre content would make you feel considerably fuller than two doughnut holes, which would make you want to eat more despite taking a lot of time and effort to chew.

A calorie is thus more than simply a calorie. To improve dietary adherence and promote fat reduction, you should also concentrate on the quality of your food.

The Macronutrient Ratio That You Can Maintain Is the Best

Although your diet's macronutrient makeup may not have a direct impact on fat reduction, it could have an impact on your capacity to follow a lower-calorie diet.

This is significant since research indicates that following a lower-calorie diet is the best predictor of weight reduction. However, most individuals find it difficult to stay on a diet, which is why so many diets fail. Tailor your macronutrient ratio to your tastes and health to maximize your chances of success on a low-calorie diet.

For instance, a low-carb diet may make it simpler for persons with type 2 diabetes to regulate their blood sugar levels than a high-carb diet.

On the other hand, those who are otherwise healthy could discover that a high-fat, low-carb diet is easier to stick to and that it makes them feel less hungry than a low-fat, high-carb diet.

Diets that prioritize consuming large amounts of one macronutrient—like fats—while consuming little amounts of another—like carbohydrates—are not appropriate for everyone.

Alternatively, you could discover that you can adhere to a macronutrient-balanced diet, which can also be successful in helping you lose weight.

Pre- and post-exercise nutrition

The foods you consume before, during, and after an exercise may have a significant impact on your mood and ability to reach your fitness objectives.

Do you ever wonder what foods are best to consume before and after going out? Or whether eating is required at all? These are crucial questions to ask since the right fuel may significantly impact your energy level, mood, and performance, which in turn can have a big impact on your likelihood of working out again.

There is no one-size-fits-all solution in the complicated realm of pre-and post-workout nutrition. It is important to note, however, that the food you consume before, during, and after an exercise may have a significant impact on your overall well-being and ability to reach your fitness objectives. (1) Food also affects how fast you recover from a workout, and for serious athletes, the timing of your post-training meal determines when you may resume your exercise regimen.

The precise advice about what, when, and how much to eat will vary greatly based on your own objectives, the kind and duration of your activity, and the time of day.

In general, it is recommended to have some kind of protein and carbs before to working exercise to maintain energy and promote muscle growth. However, meals heavy in fat or fibre should be avoided since they may lead to cramping and upset stomachs.

However, the kind of food you should consume before a 20-mile training run will vary from that of a 30-minute power walk. What you should know is as follows.

You don't necessarily need to eat anything if you exercise for less than an hour in the morning.

"Skipping the meal and having a glass of water might be the best option if you're trying to lose weight and have an easy or light workout in the morning," the author advises, explaining that this would stimulate your body to burn a higher proportion of body fat as fuel for your exercise.

Furthermore, compared to exercising later in the day, persons who work out before breakfast may burn more fat throughout 24 hours.

Is It Necessary to Refuel While Working Out?

Is it really necessary to replenish your energy during an exercise with a sports drink, gel, or gummy? For the great majority of individuals, the answer is no. Exercises lasting 60 minutes or fewer, such CrossFit, circuit training, yoga, light jogging, and pre- and post-exercise meals may be fuelled just with pre- and post-workout meals or snacks; throughout your session, you only need to drink water.

Decades of exercise science research has shown that those who engage in prolonged endurance activity, like riding or running for 60 to 90 minutes or more, do benefit considerably from mid-workout nutrition, which may postpone the onset of tiredness and enhance performance.

The International Society of Sports Nutrition recommends that after the first hour, you should try to consume 30 to 60 grams (g) of carbs per hour.

"Sports performance drinks, gels, and chews are excellent sources of carbohydrates that won't upset your stomach, but some people prefer bananas."

The Ideal Foods to Consume Following Exercise
The majority of individuals who work out for an hour or less and finish with a snack or meal that has a combination of carbohydrates and protein within a few hours after finishing their activity don't need a special recovery diet. However, certain individuals need to be more mindful of what they consume after a workout.

"Recovery nutrition" is often most crucial after strenuous strength- or endurance-training exercises (such as a 90-minute weightlifting session or bike ride) or when an athlete trains more than once in a single day.

What constitutes a nutritious post-exercise snack?

The majority of recovery snacks may include between 100 and 300 calories (more if you didn't eat much earlier in the day, and fewer calories if you had more before). But bear in mind that, if you're not an athlete and you're attempting to lose weight, your post-workout snack should probably be on the smaller side.

A few suggestions for post-workout snacks are:
- Banana slices with cottage cheese with raisins in bread.
- A hummus-topped whole-wheat tortilla.

- Simple Greek yogurt paired with honey and walnuts.
- Flavored kefir
- Crackers made with whole wheat, cheese, and dried figs.
- A couple of eggs, fruit, and toast

It's crucial to consume a healthy supper within two hours after working out in addition to this post-workout snack.

Extra for women who are over 40

As women approach their 40s, their nutritional demands shift to reflect the many physiological changes that accompany this stage of life. Everybody makes an effort to eat healthily, exercise, and follow other excellent habits. Taking specific nutritional supplements is another wise preventative health measure to assist general well-being. The top 8 supplements for women over 40 are listed below.

MEDICATION SUMMARY FOR WOMEN ABOVE 40

While whole food vitamins and minerals cannot be replaced by multivitamins, they may help close any gaps that may occur more often as we age.

The women's multivitamins you choose should be tailored to your age group. For instance, one that is high in iron, which is essential for menstrual women, and B vitamins, which encourage energy.

Multivitamin for Women

FATTY ACIDS OMEGA-3 FOR WOMEN OVER 40

DHA, EPA, and ALA are examples of omega-3 fats, along with their precursors. Because of their significant role in brain and eye function, low levels of omega-3 fatty acids may be linked to depression. Additionally, omega-3s may benefit the health of the joints, digestive system, and cardiovascular system.

Seafood and fish are the richest sources of EPA and DHA, although walnuts, chia, flax, and hemp seeds are also good sources of ALA. However, the amount of ALA that is transformed into EPA and DHA is rather low. It is recommended by health organizations that individuals take 500mg to 1000mg of EPA and DHA each day. Eating 4-6 meals a week that include fatty fish (such as mackerel, salmon, and herring) would be necessary to reach this objective. If you're not a frequent fish or seafood eater, consider including an omega-3 supplement in your regimen. While krill or fish oil is used in many, vegan-friendly algae oil is also used in others.

BIBOTICS

Probiotics are a kind of bacteria that naturally exist in your body and may help with digestion and immunity in women over 40. They support the upkeep of a thriving microbial ecosystem.

Numerous variables, including stress, food, and antibiotic use, may affect gut flora. Studies indicate that maintaining a balanced gut microbiota is crucial for bolstering immunological, neurological, and digestive systems.

Fermented foods including tempeh, miso, kefir, sauerkraut, and kimchi naturally contain probiotics. If these meals aren't something you eat often, think about taking a probiotic supplement. For maximum benefit, look for a broad-spectrum probiotic as opposed to a single-strain one.

Calcium and vitamin D

To maintain strong teeth and bones, one must consume enough amounts of calcium and vitamin D. Together, they are am,ong the greatest vitamins for women, particularly those over 40.

Since vitamin D is produced by our skin when it is exposed to direct UV radiation, vitamin D is also known as "the sunshine vitamin." But most of us don't spend enough time outdoors daily to generate the necessary amounts of vitamin D. Although fatty fish, UV-treated mushrooms, and other foods fortified with vitamin D are the main sources of vitamin D, many of us also don't get enough of it to fulfill our requirements. Foods high in calcium include dairy products, almond milk, legumes, leafy greens, and tofu with a calcium set.

To increase and maintain bone mineral density, one must consume enough vitamin D. Additionally, taking vitamin D supplements on a regular basis offers nutritional assistance for maintaining normal blood calcium levels. It's crucial for women to obtain adequate calcium because as they age, their bodies' ability to absorb it declines, weakening their bones.

Regarding the subject of how much vitamin D a woman should take daily, have your levels evaluated before starting a supplement so you can determine the right dosage. Seek for supplements containing vitamin D3 (cholecalciferol), since they have a higher absorption rate than those containing vitamin D2 (ergocalciferol).

If you can locate a mild calcium supplement that contains both vitamin K and vitamin D3, as some research indicates, it may increase the effectiveness of the other two elements.

Chapter Three

Meal preparation and recipe

Meal Prep is a very important aspect of body building in woman, without a good MP, you might not be able to achevé your goal. Follow thé following:

- Select both starchy and non-starchy veggies, as well as dark green, red, and orange beans and peas.
- Consume a range of fruits.
- Make grains a part of your diet every day.
- Consume only low-fat or fat-free dairy products.
- Consume protein with every meal.
- Make use of healthful oils like olive oil.

Women over 40 years who are of average height, healthy weight, and moderate exercise level should follow this example meal plan.

Meal / Food	Weight / portion size	Food group and number of serves
Breakfast		
Wholegrain cereal for breakfast paired with low-fat milk	60g cereal 1 cup (250ml) low fat milk	2 grain served, 1 milk/yoghurt / cheese Serve
Low fat yogourt	100g yogourt	½ milk/yoghurt /cheese serve
Morning break		
Coffee with milk	200 ml small Coffee	¼ milk/yoghurt /cheese serve

Lunch		
salad and chicken with Sandwich Apple	40g of two-slice bread, chicken One teaspoon margarine and one cup of mixed vegetables 1 medium	2 grain serve ½ meat and/or alternatives serve, 5g unsaturated spread (½ serve), 1 végétale serve 1 fruit serve

Afternoon break		
30g unsalted nuts	30g	1 meat and/or

		alternatives serve
milk and Coffee	Coffee 200ml small	¼ milk/yoghurt /cheese serve
Evening meal		
Pasta with minced meat and Red kidney beans, tomato, and green salad dressed with vinegar and olive oil	one cup of prepared pasta 65g cooked minced meat Half a cup kidney beans one and a half medium tomatoes	two servings of grains One serving of beef or an alternate One-half serving of vegetables Half a veggie dish

	One-half onion two cups of salad, mostly green leafy vegetables Two tsp unsaturated oil	two servings of veggies Two servings of 14g unsaturated oil)
Evening snack		
Yoghurt with reduced fat and plums	100g yogourt 1 cup stewed plums	One serving of fruit Serve ½ milk, yoghurt, or cheese.

Strategies for meal planning

Whatever your preferred eating pattern, a meal plan may be a great resource to help you make informed nutritional decisions. Discover the fundamentals of "how to meal plan" and peruse our well thought-out, accredited diet programmes for a range of objectives. There is no one-size-fits-all approach to nutrition and diets, so feel free to customise your own meal plan.

Keto diet schedule

A ketogenic, or "keto," meal plan is an eating style that is often extremely rich in dietary fat and very low in carbs. Around 75% of your calories on most ketogenic diets come from fat, 5% from carbs, and 20% from protein.

Although, there are some evidence to support this eating pattern's ability to aid in weight reduction, experts caution that it is an extremely restricted diet that is not suitable for everyone.

Juicing to gain muscle mass

Tart Cherry Strawberry Juice as Muscle Protector

One green apple

around half a cup of strawberries

Two cups of pitted tart cherries

two celery sticks

half a cucumber, sliced

half a lemon, peeled

Tart cherry juice has been shown by researchers to help avoid the damage that intensive exercise causes to muscles. Additionally, a recent research found that before a three-day race, cyclists who drank concentrated Montmorency sour cherry juice had lower levels of inflammation and oxidative stress than other competitors. This strawberry-cherry juice will thus benefit all athletes, including bodybuilders who work out hard and riders who spend hours riding mountain bikes. For best results, drink this juice before working out.

Tomato Basil Juice: A Powerful Muscle Builder

Two big, juicy tomatoes

Half a handful of basil

One full bunch of spinach

Half a lemon, peeled

Half a lime, peeled

The Purifier: Watermelon and Apple Juice

- 1 1/2 cups watermelon, or about two slices that are 1/2 inch thick.
- One apple
- Half a lemon, peeled

- A quarter-inch-long piece of ginger

The Revitaliser - Swiss Chard Leafy Green Juice

- 5–6 leaves of Swiss chard
- Two large handfuls of spinach
- One bunch of basil
- One green apple
- Two celery stalks
- Half a bulb of fennel
- One cucumber

The Apple-Grapefruit Juice Fat Burner

- One apple (choose a delicious apple such as Red Delicious or Royal Gala)
- One big, peeled grapefruit
- Six or seven mint leaves
- 2 sticks of celery

Snacks and Meal

More than 40? Dietitians Suggest These Are The Greatest Foods To Eat Every Day.

It's important to have these wholesome foods on your plate!

Foods high in calcium
Shutterstock
The likelihood of having many chronic conditions rises as you get older. Your body starts acting and reacting differently than it did when you were younger. For instance, cellular damage may cause your organs not to perform as well, and difficulties impacting many organs at once are seen.

It's enough to state that as you approach your fourth decade, you'll need to take on even more healthy behaviours to prevent diseases like osteoporosis, cardiovascular disease, Type 2 diabetes, arthritis, back pain, and vision issues, among others.

What's the greatest approach to look after yourself better?

You guessed it: maintaining a healthy, balanced diet. Deficits in some nutrients, such calcium, may cause osteoporosis, back discomfort, and muscular weakness. Conversely, an abundance of nutrients—even those deemed "healthy"—may cause one to gain too much weight, which can then cause obesity, hypertension, and other conditions.

The key to eating healthily for those in their forties is to follow this recommendation: "a diet focused on anti-inflammatory ingredients and antioxidants. Its really important to help prevent and reverse chronic conditions and illnesses."

Start with this tasty selection of meals that are appropriate for over-40-year-olds.

Berries: According to Shutterstock, antioxidants abound in berries including blueberries, strawberries, raspberries, and blackberries. Additionally, they contain a wealth of vitamins A and C, which may help prevent inflammation from causing wrinkles and other skin damage.

Thus, berries are beneficial to both your internal and external health. Cell health is maintained by antioxidants by reducing the harmful oxidation process that occurs inside cells.

Best also emphasises the nutrient-dense nature of blueberries, which means they are rich in nutrients and low in calories.

"Just one cup of blueberries contains 4 grammes of fibre and almost 25% of the RDI for vitamin C," according to her. Vitamin C is crucial for health, while fibre helps prevent belly fat and adds to the sense of fullness.

Seeds and nuts

Shutterstock

Over 40, nuts (walnuts, almonds, and pistachios) are crucial, as are flax, chia seed, and sunflower seeds. "Although vitamin E is an antioxidant that may strengthen our immunity and help us fend off infections, omega-3 fats found in nuts and seeds also contribute to the elasticity of our skin as we age."

"Walnuts are an organic source of essential nutrients that promote general health; a research found that women who consume walnuts and other nuts in their middle years are more likely to be in good health and wellbeing as they age.

Consuming walnuts may also aid in maintaining normal blood pressure, which is important to control over 40 years since high blood pressure raises the risk of heart disease, the leading cause of death in the United States.

Saturated Fish

"Fatty fish, such as salmon, tuna, and sardines are rich sources of omega-3 fats, which have been shown to reduce inflammation in ageing skin," Mitri explains. "They also keep your brain sharp, and may even have the potential to reduce the risk of Alzheimer's later in life."

Green leafy vegetables

"Leafy greens (such as kale and spinach) contain high levels of anti-aging vitamins, minerals, and fibre that may protect our cells and DNA," . "You can enjoy leafy greens raw in a salad, or sauteed with garlic and a drizzle of olive oil to get your daily dose."

In addition to being high in calcium and vitamin C, leafy greens lower the incidence of osteoporosis and maintain healthy bones with age.

Avocado

"Avocados are rich in heart-healthy fats, are anti-inflammatory, and support youthful skin," "Because of the healthy fat content, they are also satiating and can help with weight control."

Once again, hormone changes after 40 raise the risk of cardiovascular disease; avocados may help maintain a robust ticker.

Foods rich in protein

Shutterstock

"Including protein at every meal and snack is smart at any age, but especially for those 40 and older since we begin to lose muscle mass as early as our 30s," Kleiner states. "Eating heart-healthy protein throughout the day—along with strength-training—can help preserve muscle mass."

Make sure to include protein into your meals at breakfast (eggs, smoked salmon and crab are excellent options), lunch (think salad with beans, prawns or scallops), snacks (like sugar-free jerky) and supper (think lean proteins like grilled chicken and salmon).

Meal Planning and Protein Management
How to Prepare Meals.
Preparing your meals or dishes ahead of time before you intend to consume them is known as Meal Prep. Due to its ability to save a significant amount of time and money, it is quite popular among those with hectic schedules. Meal planning is a vital strategy for dieters,

particularly those following the Ideal Protein diet, to optimise their weight loss, stave off boredom, and stay on track towards their goals and beyond into maintenance.

You may fulfil your daily dietary objectives by ensuring that the portions in your meals are proper by preparing them in advance. Additionally, it keeps you from choosing unhealthy foods like prepared meals or takeaway, particularly when you're under pressure or too exhausted to cook.

Over time, meal preparing may lead to more interesting and nourishing meal selections since it necessitates making food decisions in advance.

Meal prep may be done in a lot of ways, and not all of them call for spending a whole Sunday afternoon preparing meals for the next week.

You may choose the approach or ways that work best for you.

What Advantages Does Meal Planning Offer?

Making enough food for a week could appear to take up a significant portion of your weekend. However, there are a few other ways to prepare meals, so you don't have to spend the whole Sunday night in the kitchen. There's always going to be one that suits you.

These are typical methods for meal preparation: Cooking a meal in big quantities and then splitting it into smaller parts to freeze and eat over the course of the next several weeks is known as batch cooking. These might be excellent choices for supper or lunch.

Meals that may be fully prepared in advance and then refrigerated until needed for consumption are known as make-ahead meals.

This may be a good technique for evening dinners.

Meals that are portioned out separately: Prepare fresh meals and divide them into pieces that may be refrigerated and consumed over the course of the next several days. This method works well for maintaining your portion sizes and may be used to fast lunches.

Ingredients that are ready to cook: Gathering all the components for a particular dish ahead of time, washing, dicing, and storing them to cut down on kitchen time.

The best meal prep technique for you will rely on your daily schedule and nutritional objectives.

Make-ahead breakfasts, for instance, may be a great way to streamline your daily routine. If you follow Ideal Protein, making a batch of zucchini oatmeal muffins or omelette muffins might be the difference between having a successful start to the day and missing breakfast because of time constraints. Additionally, folks who are busy in the evenings will benefit greatly from having meals prepared in bulk and stored in the freezer.

Depending on your unique circumstances, you may also mix and match the meal preparation strategies. It's a good idea to start with the method you like the most and progressively test out different options to see which one works best for you.

In a nutshell, meal prep may be done in a variety of ways depending on your daily routine, tastes, and objectives. Cooking large quantities of food to be chilled, preparing whole meals to freeze for later, and preparing individual servings to customise are a few of them.

Five Easy Steps for a Successful Meal Prep

Preparing meals might seem difficult, particularly if you're new to the process. However, it's not necessary. To meal prep like a master, follow these five simple steps:

Step 1: Make a meal prep plan

They believe that the secret to success is preparation. Especially when following a diet, a little advance preparation may make all the difference in how well your meals turn out. Meal planning not only makes cooking simpler, but it also benefits your health. People who meal plan are more likely to eat healthier foods and are less likely to be obese, according to a 2017 research.

The following are the most crucial factors to think about while organising your meals:
First things first: schedule the time you want to cook your meals.

One of the most important aspects of meal preparation is deciding when to cook.

This time is crucial since you could already be really busy taking care of your family, your job, your school, your home, and yourself.

Creating meals from scratch each day is just another difficult chore to add to your extensive to-do list.

The fact that meal planning just requires a minimal amount of time each week is its strongest feature. Any day or days that are most convenient for you may be chosen!

A lot of folks find that buying the items the day before and meal prepping on a Sunday evening works best. There are other practical methods to complete your shopping, such shopping and delivery services like InstaCart or free grocery store pickup services.

Why do most individuals find Sundays to be productive?

Sundays are ideal since most individuals tend to have a bit more spare time on that day. Sunday dinner preparation also helps you get ready for the workweek. It will assist you in getting off to a good start and provide you with a boost of energy to go through the week.

The most important thing, however, is to choose a time that works for you. Meal prep will become second nature if you approach it as a need, and you'll start to see those amazing benefits right away.

Second, decide how many and what sort of meals to eat.

It might be challenging to decide how many meals to prepare and what should be served at each meal.

It's crucial to decide which meal prep techniques work best for you and what dishes you want to make.

To determine how many breakfasts, lunches, and dinners you'll need for the next week, you need also look at your calendar.

You can find great resources for meal planning, ideas for meals, and even apps that will assist you with the preparation process. Adding a couple extra lunch and supper ideas can help provide variety, as most folks honestly go through ten different ideas every day. As it qwas previously indicated, combining different approaches—such as preparing meals fresh and freezing them—can aid in the development of flexibility and diversity.

Don't forget to account for the occasions when you may dine out of the house, such as on dates, at brunch with friends, at meetings over lunch, or at work dinners.

It's a good idea to start with a few recipes that you are already acquainted with and know you appreciate when picking what to cook. Your food planning will be facilitated by this familiarity.

It is best not to stick to a single dish for the whole week since not having a variety of foods may lead to boredom, hinder your body's ability to absorb all the nutrients it needs, and even hinder your diet's success.

Rather, go for dishes that use both new and well-known vegetables cooked in a variety of ways.

When you go into phases two and three of the Ideal Protein Diet, you should include complex carbs like quinoa, sweet potatoes, and legumes. Including a vegan or vegetarian dish in the mix and using foods high in Ideal Protein, such soups, to satisfy your protein needs are two more excellent ways to add variation to your diet.

Sources of protein include tofu, sardines, wild salmon, eggs, and chicken. For further suggestions, go to your list of permitted proteins.

Broccoli, spinach, kale, cucumbers, ginger, pepper, Brussel sprouts, cabbage, cauliflower, garlic, eggplant and zucchini are examples of non-starchy vegetables.

Avocado, normal, and extra virgin olive oils, as well as coconut oil, are examples of unsaturated vegetable oils.

Additions: Herbs, spices, salt, and pepper

You should also include grains and starchy vegetables such as quinoa, brown rice, wild rice, sweet potatoes, plantains, maize, pumpkin, pasta, buckwheat and squash if you're not following a low-carbohydrate diet or Ideal Protein Phase 1.

Regarding a Morning Meal:

Many individuals like to have breakfast in tiny quantities. It's a good idea to have a nutritious breakfast unless you're performing intermittent fasting, since this will sustain your energy and hunger throughout the day. It's a common misconception among dieters that once they start eating, it will be an uncontrollably large day. Breakfast eaters are less likely to overindulge in food or reach for snacks later in the day. Giving your body what it needs when it needs it is a wonderful way to avoid storing fat since your metabolism is at its highest in the morning.

To stay satisfied for longer, make sure you include enough amounts of protein, fiber-rich foods, and healthy fats in your diet.

For a meal at lunch or dinner:
Protein should make up 25% of your container; starchy vegetables or grains should make up another 25%; and salad greens or non-starchy veggies should make up the remaining 50%.

When portioning food, you may also use your hand as a guideline. The size of your hand would be a good representation of your protein intake if you were eating meat, fish, or poultry. The size of your fist will be an adequate serving for starchy vegetables or cereals. Low in calories, leafy greens and non-starchy vegetables are high in vitamins and minerals. You may add as much as you want to the remaining space in the container.

You may include healthy fats into your meal by using oils in your cooking or in salad dressings. Nuts, peanuts, avocados, and fatty salmon are additional excellent sources of beneficial fats.

For a lunch or dinner meal in Phase 1:

Half of your container should be filled with permitted veggies, 25% with your permitted protein, 25% with green salad, and a little amount of permitted oils, such as olive oil.

After you're at maintenance, 45–65% of your daily calories should come from carbs, 10–35% from protein, and 20–35% from fat, according to health experts. Meal portioning will assist you in achieving this breakdown. Just by glancing at your meal container, you should be able to prepare a meal that is nutritionally balanced. Furthermore, complex maths or the use of a calculator are not required.

Choose your recipes and begin cooking in step four.

Here are a few delectable dishes that you may wish to try:

Recipes for non-starchy vegetables

Sous Vide Broccoli

Vegetables Roasted in an Italian Oven

Roasted Vegetables in Italy

(If following phase 1 of Ideal Protein, omit potatoes.)

Roasted Vegetables in a Rainbow

Veggies Roasted in a Rainbow

Seasoned Vegetables with Garlic

Garlic-infused Steamed Vegetables

Recipes for proteins

Baked Breasts of Chicken

Baked Breasts of Chicken

Salmon Baked in Cedar Easy Way

Salmon Baked in Cedar Easy Way

Easy Drumsticks of Broiled Chicken

Easy Drumsticks of Broiled Chicken

Simple Roast Beef

Recipe for Ideal Proteins Chicken Fajita Rollups

Baked Fajita Roll-Ups with Chicken

Low-carbohydrate Ceviche

Ceviche

Pan Chicken and Veggies with Ideal Protein

Pan-fried Chicken with Veggies

A salad of cauliflower

Potato and Cauliflower Salad

Fried rice with cauliflower

Rice with Cauliflower Stir-Fry

Pasta with Olive Oil Hearts of Palm

Pasta with Olive Oil Hearts of Palm

salad with jicama

Salad Jicama

Pasta-Salad Rotini

Carb-free Egg Muffins

Muffins with eggs

Perfect Oatmeal Protein Zucchini Muffins

Zesty Oatmeal Muffins

Recipes using whole grains or starchy vegetables (ideal additions to the Phase 3 diet for protein)

One easy approach to prepare things in large quantities without spending a lot of time or effort is to roast them.

Step 2: Safely Prepare, Store, and Warm Foods
Many individuals overlook the crucial aspect of meal preparation that is food safety.

Food poisoning, which affects over 9.4 million Americans annually, may be prevented by preparing, storing, and reheating meals at the proper temperature.

Ways to Cut Down on Cooking Time

Meal preparation reduces cooking time, which is one of the key benefits for those who detest spending hours in the kitchen.

Here are some suggestions to shorten the time you spend cooking.

Maintain a Regular Timetable

Meal preparation requires adherence to a regular schedule. Establishing a fantastic routine will be made possible by knowing precisely when to prepare your meals and go grocery shopping.

You have complete control over the meal prep timetable. Just be sure it works with your weekly schedule. Making decisions will be simpler if you set up certain times and stick to them. This will free up your mind for other crucial matters.

Make the Correct Recipe Combination Selections

You may increase your cooking efficiency by selecting the appropriate recipes to use together.

To save time, choose dishes that can be prepared in a pressure cooker, oven, or crockpot using a variety of cooking techniques. You can't create as many meals at once and your meal prep time will increase if many recipes call for the same cooking appliance, such as an oven.

Taking this into account, it is essential when selecting meals to prepare ahead of time or thinking about cooking in bulk.
It's a good idea to choose one oven dinner and up to two cooktop meals at once, such as a soup, stir-fry and baked veggies.
After that, you may add meals to the mix that don't need cooking, such salads.
Set Up Your Cooking and Preparation Times
You will save a tonne of cooking time if your process is well-planned.

Starting with the meal that takes the longest to prepare is a smart approach to arrange your prep and cook timings. Usually, this is the dish or soup that is baking. After that dish is cooking, you may concentrate on the others.

Since you can simply create the cold meals while the other dishes are cooking, prepare them last.

Before you begin cooking, double-check the ingredients for each dish to save even more time. It is thus possible to chop the whole amount required at once if two or more recipes call for sliced onions or julienned peppers.

Your workflow may be simplified by using automated equipment, such as a pressure cooker or slow cooker.

Make a list of things to buy.
Grocery shopping may be a huge time waster.

Make sure you have a thorough grocery list organised according to your supermarket sections if you want to cut down on the amount of time you spend grocery shopping. This will expedite your shopping since you won't have to go back to an area you've already visited.

Using a food delivery service or going to the grocery store just once a week are two further strategies to cut down on the amount of time you spend shopping.

The saying "fail to plan, plan to fail" is still applicable. The secret to success on any diet, but particularly on Ideal Protein, is meal preparation.

Additionally, it may help you avoid eating less nutrient-dense fast food options and instead consume nutrient-dense, healthful meals while also saving money. Meal prep may include preparing whole meals in the refrigerator, making big amounts of food to freeze, or a combination of methods that work best for your time, preferences, and nutrition objectives. Figure out a system that works for you and set up one day each week to organise, buy for, and prepare your meals.

Chapter Four

Hormone Regulation and Menopause

Hormone production, including that of estrogen, progesterone, and testosterone, may decline with age. Hormonal imbalances brought on by this drop may result in mental and physical changes as well as health issues.

Pre-menopause, perimenopause, menopause, and post-menopause are the four major life periods during which women are most impacted by hormone reduction. A woman's body finds it more difficult to maintain the right balance and management of hormones as she moves through each stage.

Personalized hormone replacement treatment is intended to assist you in achieving the highest level of health and well-being at Balance Hormone Centre in Norman, Oklahoma.

Unbalanced hormone levels might have detrimental effects if not properly managed.

Handling the symptoms of menopause

Do you have symptoms associated with menopause? Take a look at these five shrewd suggestions for managing your symptoms and regaining your sense of self-worth.

Engage in regular exercise.

One of the finest things you can do for your health while going through menopause is to exercise. It helps with weight loss, circulation, stress reduction, and the annoyance of hot flashes and night sweats.

Almost every day of the week, 30 minutes of moderate-intensity exercise may help you wave goodbye to mood swings and exhaustion. Go for a jog, a stroll, a bike ride, or a dip in the pool.

Consume a balanced diet.

Maintaining a balanced diet is essential to controlling the symptoms of menopause. Make sure to eat a lot of fruits, vegetables, and nutritious grains to fill you full. Steer clear of processed meals and red meat. Drink plenty of water to stay hydrated instead of sugar-filled beverages.

Your hot flashes and exhaustion may be greatly reduced by eating a balanced diet and avoiding harmful foods.

Lessen Tension

During this time, try to find methods to de-stress and unwind since stress may exacerbate menopausal symptoms. To control your stress levels, try yoga, meditation, and deep breathing.

Spend time with friends and family, indulge in a sport or activity you like, get lots of restful sleep, or just relax with a hot bath to show yourself some love. Stress may be decreased by engaging in relaxation exercises.

Steer clear of triggers

Menopause symptoms might be brought on by certain factors. These include nicotine, alcohol, caffeine, and spicy meals. You may be able to lessen your symptoms if you can stay away from certain causes. Another alternative is to speak with a doctor about prescription drugs that might help you control menopausal symptoms.

Oestrogen therapy may ease the discomfort caused by hot flashes. When taken within ten years following your last menstrual cycle or before the age of sixty, the benefits probably exceed any possible hazards.

Make time to sleep.

For women going through menopause, getting enough sleep is crucial because it helps control hormone levels, enhances mood and cognitive function, and lessens physical symptoms like hot flashes. In addition to strengthening your immune system and reducing weariness, good sleep helps. Make an effort to get 7–8 hours of good sleep every night.

With any assistance, easily navigate menopause Taking care of menopausal symptoms doesn't have to be a daunting undertaking. It just got a lot simpler with these five suggestions. When going through this change, make sure you get enough rest and exercise to maintain your health.

Seek assistance if you're feeling overwhelmed without holding back. Make an online appointment or give us a call at Balance Hormone Centre if you need further help controlling your menopausal symptoms. We'll put together a strategy just for you. Together, let's strive for a happier, healthier you.

Changes in hormones during menopause
The menopause is the end of menstruation permanently brought on by a decrease in ovarian follicular activity. The onset of the endocrine, biochemical, and clinical aspects of the impending menopause is signaled by the menopausal transition. The start of menstruation irregularities is a frequent first indicator. The biology behind the menopausal transition includes ovarian alterations, the most notable of which is a significant reduction in

follicle counts, as well as central neuroendocrine changes. One reliable indicator of follicular activity that is not directly measured is follicle-stimulating hormone (FSH). Studies involving groups of women show that its concentration starts to rise many years before any clinical signs of impending menopause, especially in the early follicular phase of the menstrual cycle. Declining levels of inhibin B (INH-B), a dimeric protein that represents the reduction in the number of ovarian follicles, with or without alterations in the lining granulosa cells' capacity to release INH-B, cause an increase in FSH. Up to the start of the transition, oestrogen levels either stay mostly constant or tend to increase with age. They are often well-preserved until late perimenopause, most likely as a result of the high FSH levels. Hormone levels often fluctuate significantly throughout the transition; thus,

FSH and estradiol measurements are not accurate indicators of menopausal state. Between the ages of 20 and 40, throughout the reproductive life, there is a 50% decline in testosterone concentrations. They don't alter throughout the transition and could even increase after menopause. On the other hand, dehydroepiandrosterone (DHEA) and its sulfate, DHEAS, decrease with age, independent of menopause. Menopause symptoms may be understood as essentially arising from the significant decline in estradiol, which happens during a 3- to 4-year period around the time of the last menstrual cycle. This decline is likely to have a significant role in the onset of bone mineral density reduction in late perimenopause.

Taking care of hormone imbalance to bulk up

It's beneficial to your physical and emotional well-being to work out in your living room, beloved outdoor location, or neighborhood gym. Frequent exercise improves your mood and keeps your heart healthy. Engaging in any healthy exercise can help you maintain both your mental and physical wellness.

Exercise lowers stress levels, balances hormones, and promotes muscular growth. Women who suffer from metabolic disorders or illnesses triggered by hormones might benefit from regular exercise not just for muscle building but also for hormone balancing and improved overall health.

How Do Female Hormones Impact Loss of Weight?

Although cutting calories and eating fewer sounds like the easy way to lose weight, there are additional things that might throw off any fitness and health plan.

Hormones have an impact on several essential bodily processes, such as our capacity to burn fat and experience stress or hunger. It may be more challenging to reduce weight if a hormonal imbalance develops.

Hormones, however, are not everything. Prioritizing calorie consumption and high-quality meal selection is crucial. By doing this, hormone production will remain optimum and in good health. A few hormones that influence women's ability to lose weight include progesterone, thyroid, cortisol, and oestrogen.

The ratio of calories you burn to calories you take in each day is known as a good calorie balance. You are in a calorie deficit when your intake is lower than your expenditure. This implies that you should reduce your weight; nevertheless, ladies need more time to shed fat than men do. However, you ought to see success if you maintain a healthy lifestyle. But burning calories alone won't help you remain in shape or lose weight. Hormones are mostly responsible for managing stress levels, food, and body weight.

Women who have hormonal imbalances may find it very difficult to lose weight at times. The secret to your success is maintaining hormonal balance. This takes us back to the two things you should consider if you believe your weight reduction efforts have reached a standstill.

The two main female hormones involved in controlling and losing weight are oestrogen and progesterone. They support the control of your appetite, metabolism, and eating habits.

Premenstrual syndrome, weight gain, and weariness may all be prevented by ensuring that your levels of these two hormones are appropriate for your age.

Some women may eat more calories during the luteal phase of the menstrual cycle than during the follicular phase, despite this being a normal occurrence due to hormonal fluctuations. This is how progesterone affects hunger. It might be quite difficult to start a weight reduction programme during the luteal period due to the increased appetite. Therefore, starting during the follicular period could be preferable. In the end, women's hormone impacts on their bodies are sometimes uncontrollable, but any weight reduction programme must prioritise the dietary choices and physical activity levels chosen.

Which Hormones Aid in Muscle Building in Women's Bodies?

Human growth hormone (HGH) and testosterone are the two hormones linked to increasing muscular mass and strength. These hormones concentrate on muscle development and cell division when they are delivered into circulation.

The amount of testosterone in women is around one-tenth that of males. Women may differ in this number, which may impact how quickly they acquire muscle. Resistance training doesn't significantly alter a woman's level of testosterone, but it does alter her luteal phase androstenedione levels. Regretfully, androstenedione lacks testosterone's ability to promote muscular growth.

However, HGH increases the synthesis of proteins, which in turn accelerates the development of muscles and the breakdown of fat. In women, resistance exercise raises HGH levels. Given that the release peaks during the luteal phase, it seems that HGH is the primary hormone responsible for women's muscular growth. The release of HGH increases with muscular exhaustion. Compound exercise to failure is thus an effective approach to increase muscle growth and encourage the production of HGH.

What Are the Possible Causes of Female Hormone Imbalance?

Hormonal imbalances affect all women at various times in their lives. These often happen throughout the menstrual cycle, menopause, puberty, and pregnancy. However, endocrine, glandular, environmental, and medical disorders, as well as lifestyle choices, may significantly impact a woman's hormone levels. Hormones are produced, stored, and released into the circulation by the endocrine system to support various body processes.

The following are some of the causes of hormonal imbalances:

Overwhelming stress

unhealthy eating habits

A high amount of body fat

Diabetes Types 1 and 2

inflammation of the pancreas

Environmental contaminants

infections

Thyroid overactivity or under activity

birth control pills

elevated cortisol levels

The eating disorders anorexia and others

What Adverse Reactions Can Women Have from Hormone Imbalance? When the bloodstream contains either an excessive or insufficient amount of hormones, an imbalance in hormones results. Any excess or insufficiency may have negative repercussions since they are necessary for the body to maintain a balanced, healthy state. An imbalance in insulin, steroids, growth hormones, or adrenaline may have several effects on women.

The symptoms that women experience the most often are:

Irregular period of menstruation

Unable to conceive

Changes in mood

Bowel obstructions or diarrhoea

Pain in the lower back or abdomen

Lack of sleep

Unexpected increase in weight

Low desire

Brittle skeletal structure

Rashes on the skin

The hirsute

Foods that Can Assist in Hormone Balance and Muscle Building

The foundation of every lifestyle is a healthy, well-balanced diet. Your general health depends on maintaining the proper balance of your hormones. A few foods that may aid in controlling and maintaining hormonal balance are included below.

Hormone balance may be aided by blueberries.

blueberries. They're delicious and packed with antioxidants. In addition to helping to maintain hormone balance, consuming three to four cups of this superfood every week can also enhance your heart health, eyesight, and immunity against urinary tract infections.

Broccoli is excellent for building muscle and losing weight. These are excellent for preserving hormone equilibrium. Broccoli directly affects the body's oestrogen metabolism. Sulforaphane, another compound found in broccoli, aids in detoxification, fatty liver disease prevention, and cancer prevention. They are essential for the metabolism of oestrogen. The minerals calcium, magnesium, and potassium in this superfood aid in building stronger bones and promote the development and functioning of muscles.

Almonds. These lower the chance of getting Type 2 diabetes and help control blood sugar. Although they include a fair amount of calories, they aid in lowering harmful cholesterol levels in the body.

Apples may assist with hormone balance.

These are yet another excellent antioxidant. They contain a lot of quercetin, which lowers inflammation in the body. They also lower the risk of cancer and high blood pressure. Because it is high in fibre and low in calories, this fruit is a terrific way to build muscle and reduce weight.

Avocado. It is regarded as one of the healthiest fruits because of its high fibre and good fat content. In order to gain muscle, it decreases the absorption of oestrogen and increases testosterone levels. Avocados are an essential component of any nutritious diet for fitness, but they are also a fruit that should be used in moderation due to its high-calorie content.

Pumpkin seeds. These are an excellent way to get magnesium, a fantastic mineral for reducing stress. Magnesium supports the adrenal glands in a way that is well-suited to vitamins B5 and C. In addition to promoting hormone balance and muscular development, this helps reduce stress.

Green tea may assist with hormone balance.

Verdant Tea. It increases metabolism and allows for theanine, which lessens the body's production of cortisol. Antioxidants included in green tea may help reduce inflammation and the chance of illness.

Menopause Supplements and Meditations

Hormone replacement therapy (HRT) has been the main treatment for menopausal symptoms, but many women are unable to use it or do not want to because of the health hazards.

More than 50% of women are thought to treat their problems using complementary and alternative medicine, and 60% of them believe these non-traditional approaches are a good way to get relief. These include holistic methods (acupuncture, reflexology, and homeopathy), mind-body practices (yoga, meditation, and aromatherapy), and dietary supplements (vitamins, herbs, and minerals).

The following substances may provide relief from menopausal symptoms.

Melatonin

The pineal gland naturally produces melatonin, a hormone that aids in controlling sleep-wake cycles. Taking melatonin may aid with sleep because it decreases with age and sleeplessness is a frequent menopausal symptom.

Melatonin not only promotes sleep, but tiny research demonstrated that women taking 3 mg of the hormone improved in physical symptoms related to perimenopause when compared to controls. The study also discovered that supplementing with melatonin may help stop bone loss, although additional investigation is required.

Furthermore, research that supplemented perimenopausal women with 3 mg of melatonin for six months reported substantial benefits in menopause-related sadness and thyroid function.

Vitamin D and calcium

Bone health may suffer as a result of perimenopause-related oestrogen decline. It's critical to have enough calcium and vitamin D in particular, as well as other vitamins and minerals, to maintain healthy bones.

For women aged 18 to 50, the recommended daily allowance (RDA) for calcium is 1,000 mg. The RDA is increased to 1,200 mg after age 50. You may consume foods high in calcium or take supplements. Green leafy vegetables, dairy and soy products, fish (especially sardines) with bones, and fortified drinks are good sources of calcium.

Getting enough vitamin D is crucial to enhance calcium absorption, regardless of whether you obtain your calcium from food or supplements. Vitamin D is naturally found in sunlight, but many people don't receive enough of it, particularly those who live in colder climates or have dark skin. While the US Institute of Medicine suggests consuming 400–800 IU on average per day, other research suggests exceeding this amount to reach the safe top range of 1000–4000 IU.

The following other minerals are crucial for healthy bones: magnesium, potassium, vitamin K, and vitamin C. Eat a lot of plant foods (particularly fruits, vegetables, and legumes) to ensure you receive enough. To make sure you're meeting all of your nutritional needs, you may also want to take a multivitamin that is appropriate for your age and gender. Additionally, studies have shown that postmenopausal women may have higher bone mineral density if they take 5g of collagen peptides daily.

Another excellent strategy to boost muscle mass and bone density—both of which tend to decline when oestrogen levels drop—is via exercise. Eat enough protein to support your muscle mass even more. For women over 50, the recommended daily allowance (RDA) for protein is greater than for younger women: 1 to 1.5 grams per kilogram of body weight (1 kilogram = 2.2 pounds). 20–25 grams should be consumed with each meal.

Chapter Five

Overcoming obstacles and maintaining motivation

There will always be ups and downs in life, and sometimes we will encounter difficulties that will put our fortitude and drive to the test. Whether it's a workplace setback, personal struggles, or outside events, staying motivated in trying times is crucial to keep going ahead. We're all having hardships these days with RIFs, the economy, and division in the globe. Here are some practical tactics to help you remain motivated and get through difficult times! I'm going to provide you with a tonne of tactics in this post! (because I'm concerned!)

Establish Specific Goals: It's critical to have a clear idea of what you want to accomplish throughout difficult circumstances. Establish measurable objectives that are in line with your values and ambitions. (SMART objectives!) Divide them into more manageable, smaller tasks so you can track your progress and maintain focus (set milestones!). You'll be more motivated to overcome roadblocks if you have a clear direction and purpose (remember your WHY!).

Develop a Positive Attitude: When confronted with obstacles, a positive attitude may help. Consider the chances for learning and development rather than concentrating on your shortcomings or pessimistic views. (Always see the glass half full!) Remind yourself to be grateful for the good things in your life and surround yourself with supportive people. Accept the power of visualization exercises and affirmations to keep your mind upbeat and confidence high. (How many times have I discussed the power of visualization and how it alters your brain with you all?

Look for Assistance: Seeking assistance from friends, family, mentors, or your coach—I'm always here for you—is crucial at trying times. Talk to trustworthy people about your thoughts and worries so they can provide support, encouragement, and new insight. (They take up separate "corners of the room" seats.) They may provide insightful advice, a sympathetic ear, and the inspiration and fortitude to go on.

Look for Yourself:Taking care of oneself is essential when things are hard. To keep a solid foundation, give your physical and mental health priority. For a mood and energy boost, eat well-balanced meals, do frequent exercise, and get adequate sleep. Engage in mindfulness practices, such as meditation or deep breathing exercises, to lower stress and improve your capacity to handle difficult situations.

Divide Work into Doable Steps: In difficult circumstances, overwhelm is often a powerful demotivator. Divide difficult activities into manageable chunks. No matter how little the milestone, acknowledge and celebrate each one to keep yourself motivated and feeling accomplished. You'll feel more driven to keep going ahead and less overwhelmed by concentrating on one step at a time. PUSH ENERGY INTO WHAT YOU CAN MANAGE.

Accept Failure as a Chance to Learn: Failures and setbacks are often companions of challenges. Reframe them as opportunities for learning and development rather than as challenges. Examine what went wrong, conclude the experience, and use the knowledge gained for the next projects. Recall that every setback puts you one step closer to reaching your objectives and that failure is a necessary step on the path to achievement.

See Your Success in Pictures: One of the best strategies for staying motivated when things become hard is visualization. Spend a few minutes every day seeing yourself accomplishing your objectives and triumphantly conquering challenges. (Like I do, exercise your best self every morning!) Picture the feelings, the sense of achievement, and the good effects it will bring into your life. You may build a mental roadmap that will motivate and propel you ahead by visualizing success.

Honour Advancement: No matter how little your development seems to be, acknowledge it and appreciate it. Acknowledge the work and tenacity it took to overcome obstacles. Give yourself a reward when you accomplish milestones and objectives. (Only nutritious incentives, please! Not an ice cream container! Rewarding yourself for your accomplishments can keep you motivated and inspire you to keep going after your goals.

Although it's not always simple, it is feasible to maintain motivation when faced with difficulties if you have the correct attitude and techniques in place. You can get through difficult times with resiliency and determination if you set clear goals, adopt a positive outlook, ask for help, take care of yourself, break things down into manageable steps, accept failure as a teaching opportunity, visualize success, and celebrate your progress. Recall that nothing, good or terrible, lasts forever and that obstacles are just transitory. However, your drive and perseverance may help you move toward a more promising and rewarding future. Continue to be inspired, remain focused, and keep going!

Typical difficulties faced by women over 40

Women's bodies change with age, and these changes might result in a variety of health problems. The most prevalent health issues impacting women in this age group range from chronic illnesses to hormone abnormalities.

The better we understand these issues, the more equipped we are to implement beneficial treatments and preventative measures to maintain our health.

Hormonal imbalances and menopause, which were previously covered.

Heart Conditions

One of the main causes of mortality for women over 40 is heart disease. The risk factors for heart disease, such as high blood pressure, high cholesterol, obesity, and a sedentary lifestyle, rise with age in women. This is also the age at which inherited heart health problems become significant to watch.

The best method to keep an eye on your risk factors is to get routine checkups, which include blood pressure and cholesterol checks. Additionally, lifestyle becomes more significant since as we age, our bodies' ability to "correct" themselves and fend off ailments that are slowly gaining ground is diminished. At this point in life, lifestyle should take precedence over worries, particularly ensuring that we exercise often and steer clear of inflammatory meals (such as sugar, salt, and unhealthy fats) and low-nutrient foods.

Bowel, cervical, ovarian, and breast cancer
Women of all ages are concerned about cancer, but as they age, their risk rises. Self-examinations and routine mammograms are essential for early breast cancer detection. It's crucial to maintain your cervical smears, fecal occult blood tests, and routine examinations, particularly if you're suffering pelvic or stomach problems.
You should see a physician if you have discomfort, lack of energy, persistent fatigue, bloating, or unexpected changes in your weight

or appetite. These are not all of the symptoms, therefore women must be aware of any changes as well as the early warning signs of common tumors. Reading up and keeping track of bodily changes might help increase the likelihood of early discovery and a favorable prognosis.

The osteoporosis

Low bone density, which increases bone fragility and fracture risk, is a feature of osteoporosis. The decrease in oestrogen levels puts women over 40 at greater risk, particularly during and following menopause. Bone health may be preserved by a diet high in calcium and vitamin D, weight-bearing activities, safe outdoor activities or the use of vitamin D supplements in colder areas, and abstaining from tobacco and excessive alcohol use.

Emotional challenges

Women over 40 are more likely to suffer from emotional problems including anxiety and sadness. These problems may be exacerbated by menopause, hormonal fluctuations, and life events such as childrearing, child relocation, or taking care of elderly parents. To deal with these problems and preserve emotional well-being, it's crucial to ask friends, family, or mental health specialists for help.

Diabetes

Gaining weight and becoming older raise the chances of type 2 diabetes. Similar to heart disease recommendations, frequent testing and lifestyle changes play a major role in prevention. Early detection of type 2 diabetes may lead to reversal; maintaining frequent blood tests, cutting down on sugar and simple carbs (like white bread), and engaging in regular exercise are excellent strategies for this.

Even if you don't have a family history of diabetes, you should still monitor your health after menopause. Feelings of fatigue, thirst, increased frequency of urination, and unexplained weight fluctuations are early indicators of diabetes.

The inability to urinate

Women over 40 may have problems with urinary incontinence, or the unintentional leakage of pee. Hormonal fluctuations, weak pelvic floor muscles, or underlying medical issues might all be the reason. You don't have to suffer in silence; there are a number of solutions that help ladies with this illness. Of course, you shouldn't put off seeing a doctor because you're embarrassed—this is a fairly frequent problem.

Thyroid Conditions

The prevalence of thyroid conditions, such as hyperthyroidism or hypothyroidism, is higher in women over 40. Thyroid issues may strike later in life, which may surprise some of you. Numerous symptoms, including exhaustion, mood swings, hair loss, and weight gain or loss, might be brought on by these disorders. Any thyroid abnormalities may be diagnosed and managed with the use of routine thyroid function testing, and therapy is straightforward and efficient.

Although women over 40 are more likely to have certain health problems, it's crucial to keep in mind that every woman's health journey is different. Preventing and treating these prevalent health issues may be greatly aided by regular exercise, a balanced diet, keeping a healthy weight, quitting smoking, and routine check-ups and blood testing.

Although women are often told to "get on with it," their quality of life counts. Always put your health first is what we always advise. Since our clinic is managed by women, we are aware of how busy women can become and that they often overlook small symptoms in favor of taking care of those close to them. You are cordially invited to make it right and make sure you're well for the people you care about as well as for yourself.

Techniques for maintaining motivation and consistency

Establish definite, attainable objectives for yourself and put them in writing. You'll be more driven and concentrated as a result.

Make a timetable: Set up a regular timetable for your tasks or hobbies. It will be simpler for you to follow your strategy and will help you develop consistency.

Employ prompts: To stay on track and remember critical tasks or deadlines, set up alerts or notifications on your device.

Divide up the work into smaller steps: Divide a big job or assignment into smaller, easier-to-manage segments. This will support you in maintaining concentration and advancing towards your objective.

Create a positive habit: Since habits are the foundation of consistency, create a good habit that advances your objectives. For instance, if you want to work out often, develop the habit of going to the gym or going for daily walks.

Be responsible for yourself: Establish self-accountability goals, such as updating a friend or mentor on your progress. This might support your motivation and goal commitment.

Steer clear of distractions: Recognise and stay away from distractions that may cause you to lose consistency and attention. TV, social media, and other time-wasting media may fall under this category.

Remain organized: To lower stress and boost productivity, keep your workplace and calendar in order. To keep organized, make use of tools like calendars, to-do lists, and productivity apps.

Remain upbeat: Remaining upbeat can help you remain consistent and motivated. Celebrate your little victories along the road and keep your attention on your development and achievements.

Review and tweak: Keep a close eye on your development and tweak your plan of action as necessary. This will ensure that you are making progress towards your objectives and help you remain on course.

Change in Mindset to Sustained Success
Accept failure rather than running from it: Learning happens more quickly the more mistakes one makes. Henry Ford started several

unsuccessful ventures before launching his vehicle manufacturing firm. If he had given up after his first attempt, how would the industrial landscape have looked? Recall that accepting failure may also make success come much faster.

Consider plenty as opposed to scarcity. Many individuals are hesitant to spend money on themselves because of the expense. However those who appreciate and trust in themselves tend to attract clients and consumers. Consider personal development as an investment in your future rather than an outlay of money.

Accept challenges. Individuals with a "growth" attitude tend to actively seek out possibilities because they understand that obstacles are opportunities waiting to be discovered.

Turn setbacks become teaching moments. There will always be roadblocks, regardless of how detailed the plan is or how well the specifics are carried out. Furthermore, who is capable of foreseeing what obstacles would arise? Rather than expending energy attempting to stop the unknown, why not just confront challenges as they arise?

Keep things in perspective. Taking advantage of unfavorable comments and harsh criticism may provide some of the finest chances for both career and personal development. To what extent do you respond to grievances raised by clients and customers?
Give up on creating new things. Rather of harboring resentment against outstanding individuals, seek to understand their methods and use them to your benefit.

Managing Obstacles and Plateaus

Understanding the reason behind any plateau—real or imagined—is crucial to breaking over it. The plateau will eventually go if our brain just requires time to assimilate new knowledge before we can proceed. But if we've reached a plateau of complacency, we overcome it by pushing ourselves and renewing our dedication to the art.

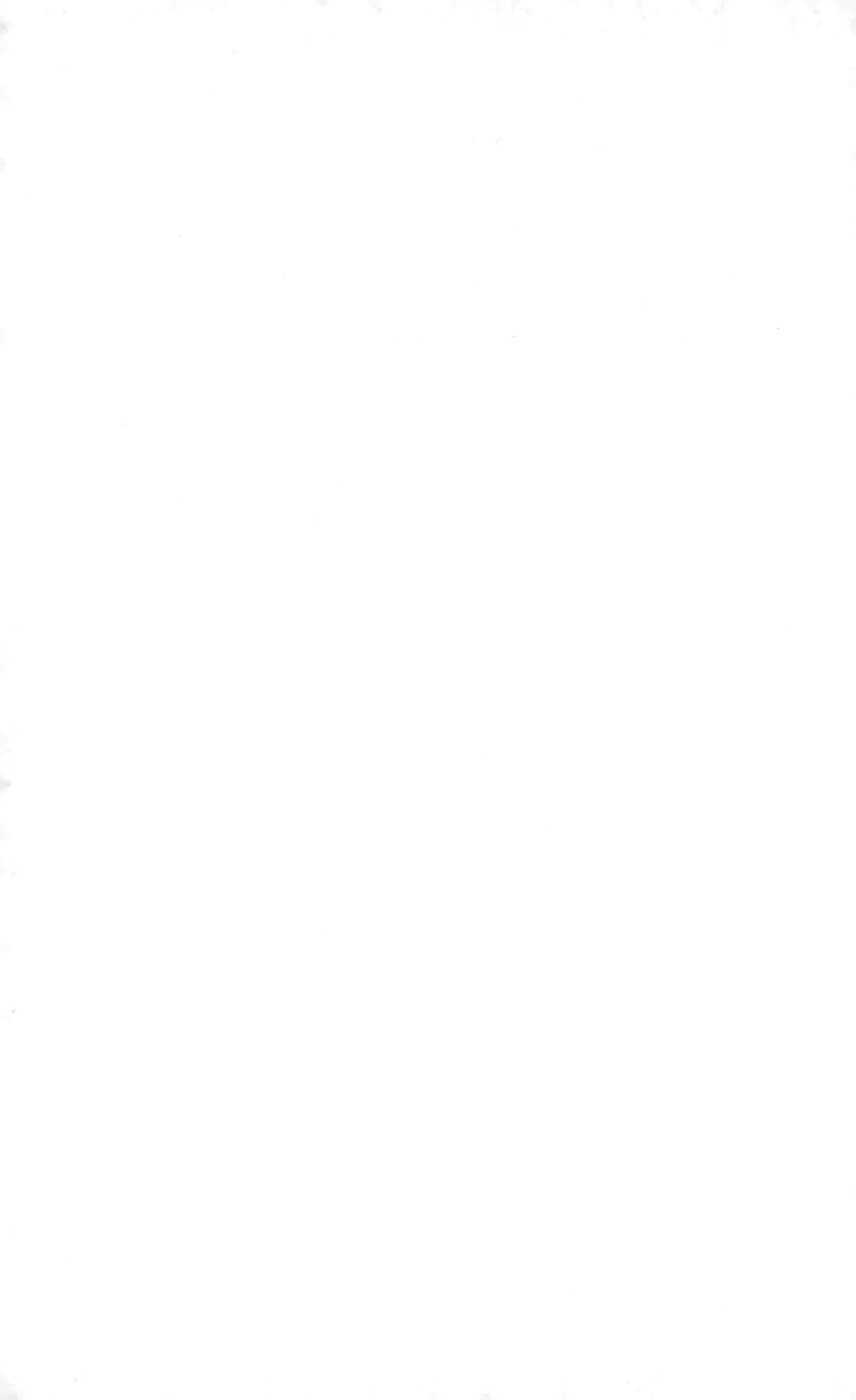

www.ingramcontent.com/pod-product-compliance
Lightning Source LLC
Chambersburg PA
CBHW070845260726

48661CB00004B/1252